Linda Bel Hadj Kacem
Chaima Ghrairi

Study of the pre-analytical phase

Linda Bel Hadj Kacem
Chaima Ghrairi

Study of the pre-analytical phase

in the anatomy and pathological cytology laboratory

ScienciaScripts

Imprint

Cover image: www.ingimage.com

This book is a translation from the original published under ISBN 978-620-6-71924-3.

Publisher:
Sciencia Scripts
is a trademark of
Dodo Books Indian Ocean Ltd. and OmniScriptum S.R.L publishing group

120 High Road, East Finchley, London, N2 9ED, United Kingdom
Str. Armeneasca 28/1, office 1, Chisinau MD-2012, Republic of Moldova, Europe
Printed at: see last page
ISBN: 978-620-2-91117-7

DR LINDA BEL HADJ KACEM

CHAIMA GHRAIRI

STUDY OF THE PRE-ANALYTICAL PHASE IN THE PATHOLOGICAL ANATOMY AND CYTOLOGY LABORATORY

TABLE OF CONTENTS

INTRODUCTION

The concept of quality in healthcare remains a universal concern, and continuous improvement is a challenge for effective care. However, compared with other areas of medical biology, quality assurance and improvement plans in pathological anatomy and cytology (PCR) are recent concepts [1].

Anatomopathological examination (AP) takes place in three phases: the pre-analytical phase, the analytical phase and the post-analytical phase. It is a decisive factor in the diagnosis, treatment, evaluation of the therapeutic effect and prognosis of diseases [2].

Most samples for AP examination are unique and irreplaceable, which is why it is necessary to provide the most accurate results possible since they have a direct impact on the patient's health [1].

Despite changes in sample handling practices, the pre-analytical phase is still the source of the most non-conformities (85% of non-conformities affecting the validity of analysis results) [1]. This prompted us to ask the question :

How can NCs that occur during the pre-analytical phase in the PCR laboratory be identified and corrected?

In response to this problem, the aim of our study is to detect NCs that occur during the pre-analytical phase in PCR and to propose corrective actions to ensure optimal improvement of this phase.

OBJECTIVES

- Identification of NCs in the pre-analytical phase in our pathological anatomy and cytology laboratory.

- Proposing corrective actions to improve the pre-analysis phase.

BIBLIOGRAPHICAL STUDY

I. Pathological anatomy and cytology laboratory

I.1-Definition

"PCA refers to the medical discipline that studies tissues and cells, using techniques based on macroscopic and microscopic morphology" [4].

I.2-Nature of the samples

PCA samples can be obtained in different ways.

I.2.a-Cytological samples

Cytology can be obtained in various ways:

• Cytopuncture: involves removing cells by capillary action using a very fine needle (25 gauges) (figure 1).

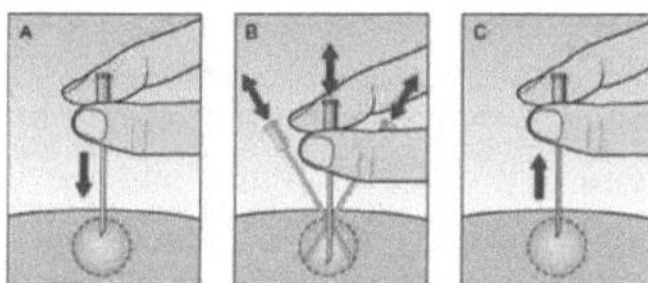

Figure 1: Cytology sampling technique (Cytopuncture)[5].

• Collection of spontaneous fluids (urine, sputum).

• Brushing, scraping, swabbing of spontaneously desquamating cells.

• Affixing a cloth to a slide.

• Puncture of fluid from ascites, pleural effusion and cysts [4].

I.2.b-Histological samples

• Biopsy: removal of a fragment of tissue for an AP examination.

• Surgical parts: complete or partial removal of one or more organs.

• Autopsy: AP examination carried out on a corpse to determine the cause or causes of death [4].

I.2.c-Extemporaneous examination

Examination requested by a surgeon during a surgical procedure while the patient is still in the operating theatre. It enables a rapid diagnosis to be made in order to guide the surgical procedure [4].

I.3-Mission of pathological anatomy and cytology

The CPA's mission is to :

- Make a diagnosis on the basis of tissues and/or cells taken from the patient.
- To evaluate the therapeutic effect during a course of treatment in order to assess the disappearance, persistence or worsening of a lesion [4].

II. Quality in the anatomy and pathology laboratory

II.1-General points

The concept of quality goes back a long way in human evolution. The concepts of quality management appeared at the end of the 19th century and the beginning of the 20th century [6].The emergence of the concept of quality was influenced by the rationalisation of work and mass production driven by Frederick Winslow Taylor and Henry Ford. At the time, quality was limited to checking the conformity of the finished product [6].In 1916, Henri Fayol set out the 5 fundamental principles of administration: planning, organising, commanding, coordinating and controlling in a book entitled Administration industrielle et générale. Control is no longer confined solely to the conformity of the finished product, but also includes an analysis of errors in the production process. production process in order to take corrective action [7].In 1947, the International Organization for Standardization (ISO) was created [6].In 1990, the ACP structure wanted to initiate an autonomous quality approach by creating the Association Française d'Assurance Qualité en Anatomie et Cytologie Pathologiques (AFAQAP). AFAQAP is a not-for-profit association. It regularly assesses and improves the quality of pathologists' practices in various areas (diagnosis, sample handling techniques and laboratory organisation) [8].

II.2-Accreditation of anatomy and pathology laboratories

Accreditation is a "procedure whereby an authoritative body provides formal recognition that an organisation is competent to carry out specific tasks" [9]. The aim of this procedure is to guarantee the reliability of examinations by means of an assessment of the competence of the CPA structure by peers who are independent of the structure to be accredited [9].

II.3-The international standards organisation

ISO is an international standards body made up of representatives of national standards organisations from 158 countries. Its aim is to produce international standards in industrial and commercial fields, known as ISO standards [10].

A standard is "a document established by consensus and approved by a recognised body, which provides, for common and repeated use, rules, guidelines or characteristics for activities or their results, guaranteeing an optimum level of order in a given context" [6].

II.3.a-ISO9001 "Quality management system" standard

ISO 9001 is a standard that defines the requirements for a quality management system.
It guarantees patients services that meet their expectations [11].

II.3.b- Standard ISO 17025 "General requirements for the competence of testing and calibration laboratories".

According to ISO, standard 17025 is an international standard that establishes the general requirements of competence for carrying out tests and/or calibrations, including sampling. It helps to increase the confidence of laboratories in providing reliable and valid test, calibration and sampling results [12].

II.3.c- ISO 15189 standard: "Laboratoires d'analyses de biologie médicale - Exigences particulières concernant la qualité et la competence" (Medical biology analysis laboratories - Particular requirements concerning quality and competence)

ISO 15189 is an international standard specific to medical laboratories. It is based on ISO9001 and ISO17025, with the aim of accrediting medical laboratories [13].

The first version was drafted in 2003, the second in 2007, then a version in 2012 and the current version is that of 2022 [14].

ISO 15189 describes the specific quality requirements and procedures to be followed in the pre-analytical phase [15].

III. Quality assurance and quality tools

Today, quality assurance is recognised as a criterion of trust. It is a global concept that focuses on the entire quality system, including suppliers and all the personnel involved in achieving the desired level of quality [1].

Quality tools include the PDCA (plan-do-check-act) method and the Ishikawa diagram.

III.1 PDCA method

The PDCA method was developed by Walter Shewhart in 1930. In 1950, the statistician William Edwards Deming represented it to Japanese industrialists in the form of a wheel known as the Deming wheel (Figure 2) [16].

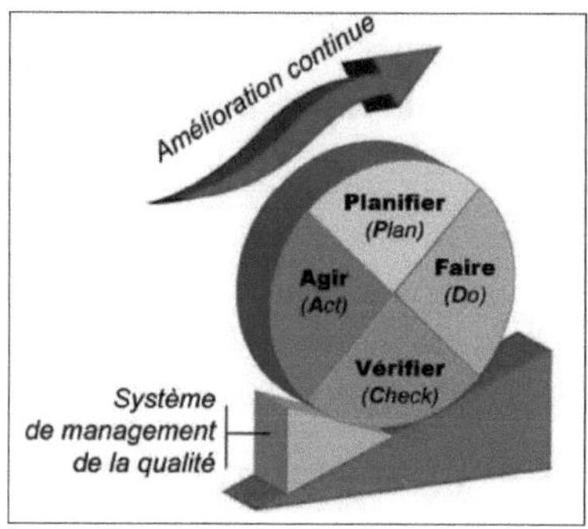

Figure 2: Deming Wheel representation [17].

It's a virtual circle divided into four parts and placed on a slope. Each quadrant is marked with a letter P.D.C.A. The idea is to repeat the 4 phases: Plan-Do-Check-Act until the desired objective is achieved.
The PDCA method stands for Plan, Do, Check and Act.

✓Plan: to plan, which consists of preparing the work to be done and the means and resources needed to achieve the objectives set.
✓Do: to do, which consists of carrying out or implementing the planned work.

✓Check: to verify that the objectives initially set have been achieved.

✓Act: Act to improve, which consists of implementing improvement actions [16].

III.2-Ishikawa diagram

The cause-effect diagram was developed by Professor Kaoru Isikawa in 1943. It is also known as the Ishikawa diagram, the 5M method (Material, Equipment, Manpower, Environment and Methods), or the fishbone diagram because of its shape (Figure 3) [18].

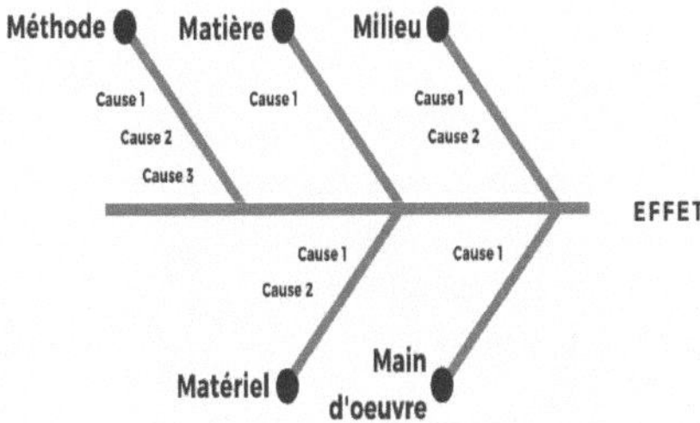

Figure 3: Representation of the Ishikawa diagram [17].

The 5M analysis makes it possible to determine the possible causes of NC in order to reduce or eliminate them. We can then determine which cause should be given priority for corrective action [18].

✓Material: This covers raw materials, supplies, data, documents, etc.

✓Equipment: This groups together the possible causes of technical support (machines, equipment, tools, etc.) and the products used.

✓Workforce: includes training, motivation, skills, organisation, etc.

✓Environment: This concerns the environment, working conditions, noise, light, etc.

✓Methods: includes work rules, procedures, operating methods, etc. [18].

IV. Stages of anatomopathological examination

The AP examination takes place in three phases (Figure 4):

The pre-analytical phase, which is the objective of our study, covers all the stages from the prescription to the actual microscopic analysis.

The phase analytical : this phase includes the reading microscopic reading and interpretation of the slides by the pathologist.

The post-analytical phase: this involves communicating the results to the doctors in charge of the patient and archiving the slides and blocks [2].

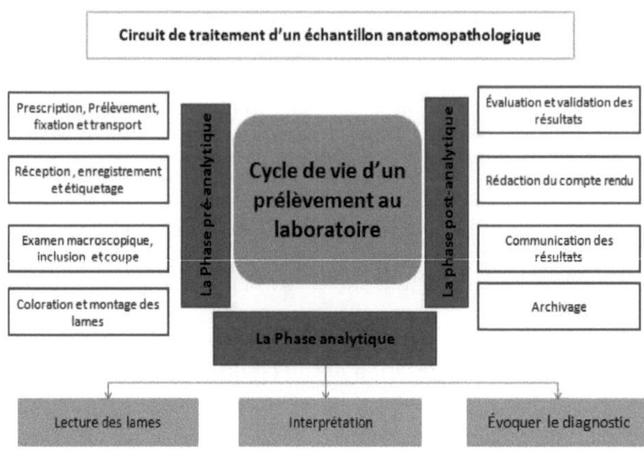

Figure 4: PCA-adapted representation of the different phases of an AP examination [19].

IV.1- Pre-analytical phase in pathological anatomy and cytology IV.1.a-Definition of the pre-analytical phase

All the stages starting with the test prescription, followed by sample collection, fixation and transport to the laboratory, reception, registration, labelling of vials and sample handling. macroscopic examination, dehydration, paraffin embedding, microtome sectioning, staining and slide mounting [1].

IV.1.b-Specificity and complexity of the pre-analytical phase

Most AP samples are unique and irreplaceable, so a standardised procedure is needed to obtain results that comply with the standards set by the laboratory [2].
This phase is very time-consuming and requires a lot of human resources, as most of these steps are manual.It is a major source of error since :

- A large part of this phase takes place outside the laboratory, so it cannot be controlled.
- It involves a number of human manipulations and interventions, including operating theatre staff, the courier, technicians, secretaries and doctors.
- Producing a slide for microscopic examination is a complex and slow process [2,3].

IV.1.c-Actors in the pre-analytical phase

Carrying out the pre-analytical phase in PCR requires skilled, competent staff (Table I) who are aware of its importance and of all the possible NCs that can influence the results of the analysis. [20]

Table I: players in the pre-analytical phase in PA [20].

Activities	People involved
Prescription	Doctor
Withdrawals	Doctor, surgeon
Fixing	Sampler, operating theatre technician, Laboratory technician
Transport	Courier, nurse, labourer
Reception	Reception staff
Macroscopic examination	Pathologist
Sample handling	Laboratory technicians

IV.2-Steps in the pre-analytical phase

The pre-analytical phase takes place in two stages, the first often outside the laboratory and the second inside the laboratory (Appendix 1) [19].The external pre-analytical phase is carried out by the prescriber, sampler and transporter, whose tasks end when the vials are received in a state that complies with the standards used by the laboratory.The internal pre-analytical phase begins with the reception of samples and ends with the mounting of slides for microscopic analysis [17].

IV.2.a-External pre-analytical phase

The external pre-analytical phase consists of a series of stages:

- **Prescription**

It is a medical procedure, carried out by qualified doctors. It must answer a clinical question and is based on good practice recommendations [17].

- **Direct debit**

Sampling is a medical procedure that involves taking a biological sample in order to obtain a precise diagnosis [4].

- **Packaging**

The samples taken are placed in bottles appropriate to their size and type [20].

- **Fixing**

Fixation is an essential step in preserving cell morphology in a state close to the living state and avoiding autolysis (the lysis of living tissue by its own enzymes). It is a definitive and irreversible stage [21].
It must be carried out immediately after the sample is taken [4].

The fixative most commonly used in histology is a 4% aqueous formalin solution. stamped [4]. For good quality fixation, :

✓The volume of formalin should cover approximately 5 times the volume of the part to be fixed.

✓Choose a bottle suitable for the size of the sample.

✓Before fixation, hollow organs such as the digestive tract and uterus should be opened and large organs sliced to facilitate penetration of the fixative [4].

✓Fixer penetration speed: Fixers penetrate tissue at different speeds and vary from one fixative to another. In general, fixatives have a penetration speed of approximately 1.0 millimetre/hour (Figure 5).
The figure below (Figure 5) shows the rate of penetration of formalin into a 25 millimetre thick liver sample. [21]

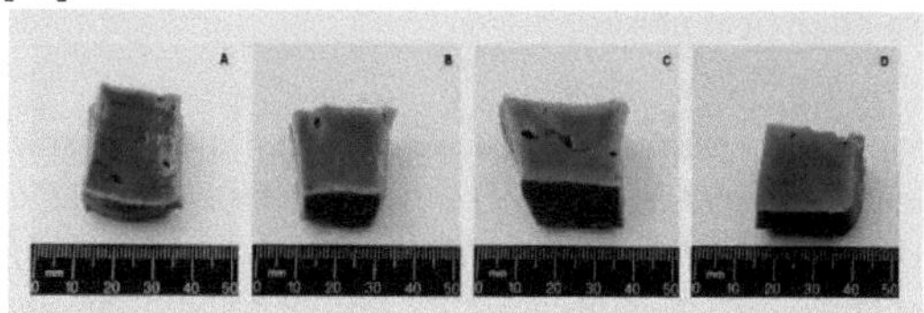

Figure 5: Penetration speed of formalin in a 25 mm thick liver sample [21].

A: approximately 0.8 millimetre penetration of fixative for one hour B: 1.2 millimetre penetration of fixative for two hours C: approximately 1.6 millimetre penetration of fixative for four hours D: 2 millimetre penetration of fixative for eight hours. Note that after eight hours of fixation, the centre of the sample remains unfixed.

✓Fixation time: this depends on the size of the sample, approximately 6 hours minimum for a biopsy and 24 to 48 hours for a surgical specimen.
✓Hydrogen potential (PH): the PH of the fixative must be close to the physiological PH and between 6.8 and 7.2 [21].

• Fixer

There are several reagents (Bouin's liquid, Carnoy fixative, etc.) that can be used to fix histological samples. The most commonly used fixative is a 4% buffered aqueous formalin solution [20].
Formalin is a chemical fixative that was used as a PCR fixative in the 1890s by Ferdinand Blum [20].
Buffered 4% formalin is obtained by diluting one part of 40% concentrated formalin with 9 parts of water or buffer. This produces a 10% formalin solution containing approximately 4% formaldehyde, an ideal concentration for fixation [21].

• Identification of samples

Each vial must have a unique identification because it represents a unique link between the patient and the examination requested.

To ensure proper identification, all vials should be labelled with the patient's first and last name and an identification number unique to each patient [22].

• **Request for anatomopathological examination**

Each sample must be accompanied by an examination request form [20]. This request must provide all the information required for the examination to be carried out correctly and for the results to be interpreted, such as :

- Patient identification: first and last name
- Patient's date of birth
- Sex of the patient
- Identification of the requesting department
- Identification and signature of the sampler
- Type of samples
- Date and time each sample was taken
- Degree of urgency if necessary
- The clinical, paraclinical and evolutionary information needed to interpret the AP sample [20].

• **Transporting samples**

The ISO 15189 standard requires each laboratory to ensure that samples are transported under optimum conditions to preserve sample integrity [15].
The carrier must comply with the time limits appropriate to the nature of the tests requested.
The carrier may be a courier, a nurse, a hospital worker or a patient [20].

IV.2.b-Internal pre-analytical phase

Various successive stages precede the AP analysis to ensure the reliability of the results.

• **Reception**

Receiving samples is an important stage in obtaining quality results. Each laboratory has a document setting out the criteria for accepting and rejecting applications [20].

It is carried out by authorised personnel who must systematically check that the information on the test request form matches the samples, to ensure that the data is correct [22].

• **Registration of examination requests**

Once the data has been assessed for conformity, the requests for AP examinations are recorded in a computer system or in the laboratory register [20].

• **Labelling**

Each sample is labelled with :

- ❖ Unique patient identification
- ❖ The bar code
- ❖ The identification number
- ❖ The type of examination (cytology or histology) [20].

• Dehydration

Dehydration consists of removing the intracellular water from the fixed tissues so that fine cuts can be made without losing the initial cellular structure at the time of cutting (sudden release of water). It is necessary to retain 2% to 3% intracellular water to facilitate cutting and avoid hardening of the part [20].

• Paraffin embedding

The paraffin embedding stage provides an external support for the tissues to facilitate cutting by the microtome and to ensure that the tissues are well preserved after cutting.
Inclusion is performed using a paraffin embedding machine. The machine must be cleaned to avoid contamination by tissue residues [22].

• Sectioning using the microtome

This step produces ribbons of cuts of varying thickness. The thickness of the sections is chosen according to the tissue and the staining required (as a general rule, 3 to 5 micrometres) [22].

• Spreading on glass slats

Spreading allows the ribbons to lie flat in a hot water bath before being collected on slides for microscopic examination [4].

• Staining and slide preparation

The routine stain for PCR is haematoxylin and eosin (HE).

HE staining reveals the nucleus and cytoplasm of cells. Haematoxylin stains the nucleus purple and eosin stains the cytoplasm pink.The stain used in cytology is the Papanicolaou stain. Papanicolaou staining highlights the nucleus, cytoplasm and presence of keratin in the cells. Haematoxylin stains the nucleus purple, Eosin Azure stains the cytoplasm pink and Papanicolaou OG6 stains cells containing keratin orange [4].
Checking staining parameters such as the time required in each staining bath, reagent concentration, quality control of solutions and bath maintenance will improve the quality of the slides obtained [20].

• Fitting the blades

Mounting the slides involves protecting the fragment by applying a coverslip to the slide using a mounting medium that must be transparent and free of any stain.

Proper mounting technique involves avoiding the presence of air bubbles by pressing gently on the coverslip with the fingers [22].

V. Management of non-conformities in the pre-analytical phase

According to the ISO9000 definition, a NC corresponds to the failure to satisfy a requirement. It may concern any stage of the PCA examination [17].

V.1-Possible non-conformities committed during the pre-analytical phase in the pathological anatomy and cytology laboratory

V.1.a-No application form or bottle

A sample without a request form or a request without a sample is a NC which prevents the analysis from being carried out.

V.1.b-Imprecise patient identification

The staff responsible for reception are often faced with examination request forms that are incomplete or have illegible handwriting (figure 6).This NC may prevent the analysis from being carried out and the results from being interpreted [23].

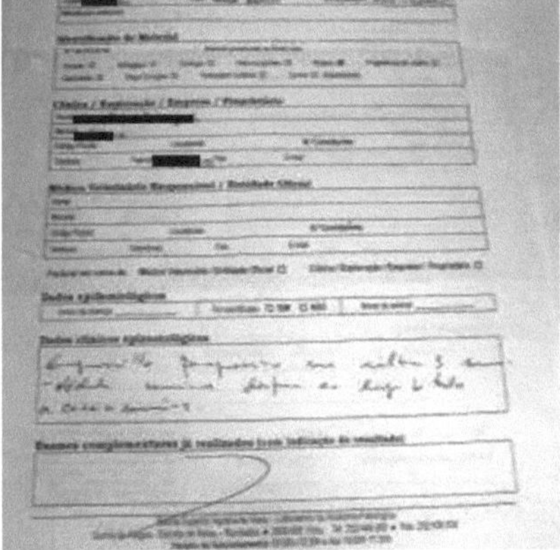

Figure 6: Example of a request form with incomplete information and illegible handwriting [23].

V.1.c-Mismatch between the patient's name on the request form and on the bottle

Discrepancies between the patient's name on the request form and the sample taken result from the fact that the staff identifying the tube are different from those taking the sample, or when the sample is sent to the laboratory before the patient's details have been checked. This NC prevents the test from being carried out [17].

V.1.d-Absence of date and time of sampling

Specifying the date and time of sampling is important, as it gives the pathologist an idea of how long the sample will be fixed or not fixed if the sample is received unfixed [23].

V.1.e-Absence of clinical, paraclinical and developmental information

In the histological and cytological study carried out by the pathologist, clinical, paraclinical and evolutionary information is very important, as it provides information concerning the patient's medical history, thethe examinations carried out and the diagnoses suggested, which can guide and help the pathologist to interpret the results. The absence of clinical information can influence the relevance of the result [22].

V.1.f-Absence of the doctor's stamp or signature

The request form must be correctly signed by the prescribing doctor if he is to assume his responsibility [17].

V.1.g-Vial identification error

Incomplete or inaccurate data on the sample label may lead to :

- Discrepancy between the results of the AP examination and the patient's clinical condition.

- Inappropriate therapeutic conduct.

- Delayed diagnosis.

Misidentification of the sample is a blocking NC [20].

V.1.h-Packaging error

NCs for sample conditioning include :

- Vial size not adapted to sample size (figure7)

- Bottle not properly closed, leading to the risk of formalin leakage and/or loss of all or part of the sample [23].

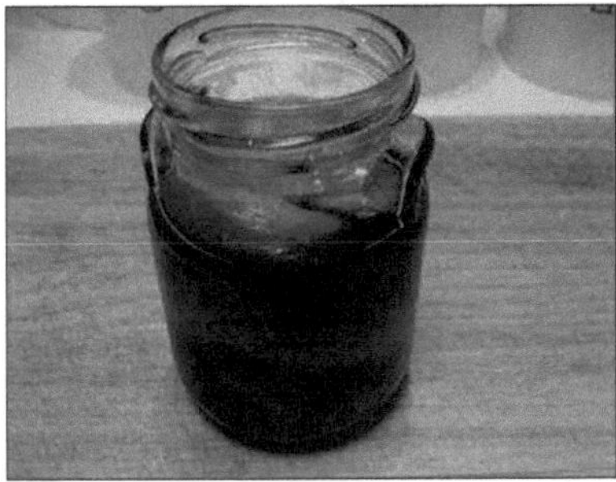

Figure 7: Example of a bottle unsuited to the size of the sample [23].

V.1.i-Inappropriate fixing

Poor fixation conditions have a direct impact on sample quality, such as :

- The absence of fixation.
- Wrong choice of fixative.
- Insufficient volume of fixative (figure 8) [23].

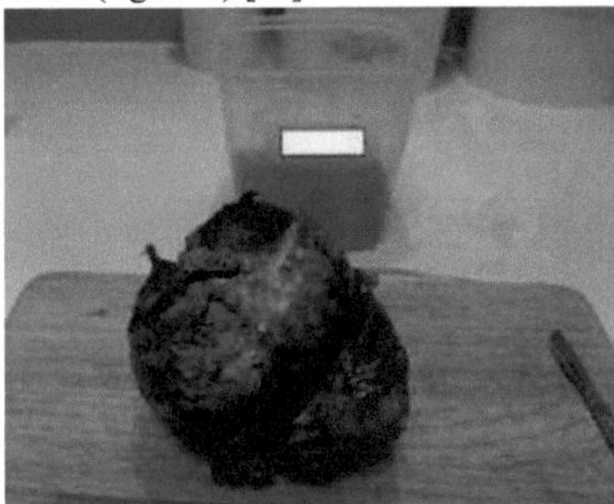

Figure 8: Volume of fixative insufficient for sample size [23].

V.1.j-Dehydration error

Excessive dehydration results in very hard fragments, which will affect the quality of the microtome section.Insufficient dehydration results in soft tissue that is difficult or impossible to cut [4].

V.1.k-Deleted identification number

If the identification number is erased from the blocks or slides, the examination will be blocked and the results will be erroneous (Figure 9) [23].

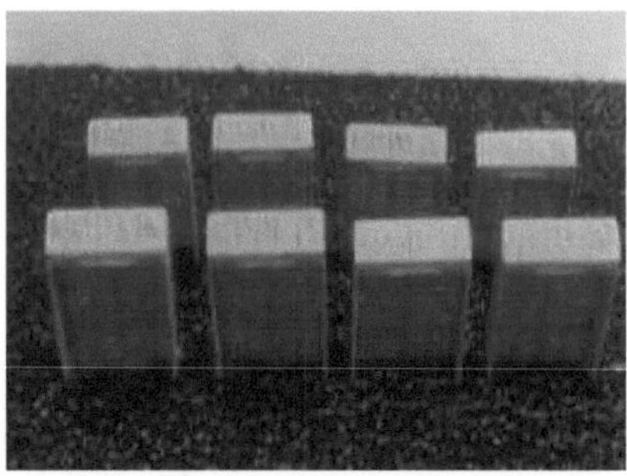

Figure 9: Deleted identification numbers [23].

V.1.l-Thick section

Thick sections will influence the microscopic reading of the slides, making it difficult to distinguish between the different structures and cells [22].

V.1.m-Colouring error

Excessive or insufficient staining of slides can make microscopic reading difficult [22].The different types of NC are summarised and represented in the following table:(table II).

Table II: Summary table of the different types of NC in PCA.

Type of non-compliance	
Blocking NC	Non-blocking NC
-No request for examination. -incorrect patient identification Discrepancy between the patient's name on the request form and the bottle Lack of relevant clinical information. -Absence of sample. Incorrect identification of vials Unsuitable fastening Dehydration error -Deleted number on block or blade	Absence of date and time of sampling. - Absence of the prescribing doctor's stamp or signature. Packaging error Thick cut Colouring error

V.2-Management of pre-analytical NC in anatomopathology

According to ISO 15189, NC control is a regulatory requirement [15]. NCs are very frequent and affect all stages of the pre-analytical process [2]. All NCs must be detected, identified, recorded and corrected [17].To improve the pre-analytical phase, the first step is for the staff in charge to record these NCs on a form called the NC form.It is not enough to detect them, but they must be corrected, by researching and analysing the causes, assessing the associated risks and establishing preventive and improvement actions.Immediate correction or treatment of CKD is the responsibility of the person who detects it, within the limits of their competence [17,19].

MATERIALS AND METHODS

I. Presentation of the study

We conducted a descriptive observational study in the PCR laboratory. The study was conducted over a period of 3 years and 5 months, from January 2020 to 27 May 2023. We began with a tour of the laboratory's various units and an observation of the daily internal pre-analytical phase in PCR.We then identified and recorded the daily NCs that reach the laboratory.Thirdly, we drew up a questionnaire (Appendix 2) for the various staff in the PCR laboratory who are involved in the pre-analytical phase. This questionnaire covered the different stages of the pre-analytical phase, staff knowledge of NCs, the frequency with which NCs are recorded and how they can be managed. It was examined by the dissertation supervisor and the head of the PCR laboratory department to validate the content so that each of these questions was formulated in a clear and easily interpretable way.

II. Inclusion criteria

We have included the different types of pre-analytical NC in our study.

III. Exclusion criteria

We have excluded from our study the different types of analytical and post-analytical NC, and NC from complementary diagnostic techniques (immunohistochemistry and molecular biology).

IV. Presentation of the anatomy and pathology department

The PCR laboratory is run by a department head assisted by unit heads. Its main activities are: conventional histopathological examination and extemporaneous examination, conventional cytological examination and molecular analyses: Polymerase Chain Reaction (PCR), sequencing, etc. and specialised additional tests: special staining, immunohistochemistry and in situ hybridisation. It receives histological samples (autopsy samples, biopsies, surgical specimens, etc.) and cytological samples (cervico-uterine smears, bronchial fluid, etc.). To carry out its tasks effectively, the PCR laboratory has a number of resources at its disposal, including premises, staff, equipment and reagents, all of which are shown below in the form of an organisation chart (figure 10).

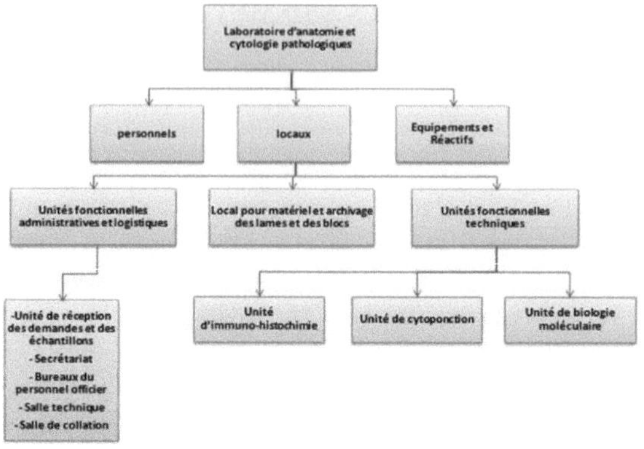

Figure 10: Organisation chart of the PCR laboratory.

V. Course of the phase pre-analytical phase at the anatomy and pathological cytology laboratory of our hospital

The daily schedule for the pre-analytical phase of cell and tissue sampling is as follows:

V.1- Acceptance

In the presence of the requesting department's courier, the samples received and the AP examination request forms (Appendix 3) were checked by verifying all the following points on the request forms and on the vials:

- The patient's identity: surname, first name, date of birth, sex.
- The date (day and time) and nature of the sample.
- The presence of the patient's clinical details.

V.2- Registration

The samples are then recorded in the laboratory's Electronic Medical Record (DMI) (figure 11) and given a unique identification number which will be transcribed onto the blocks and slides to be examined by the pathologist.

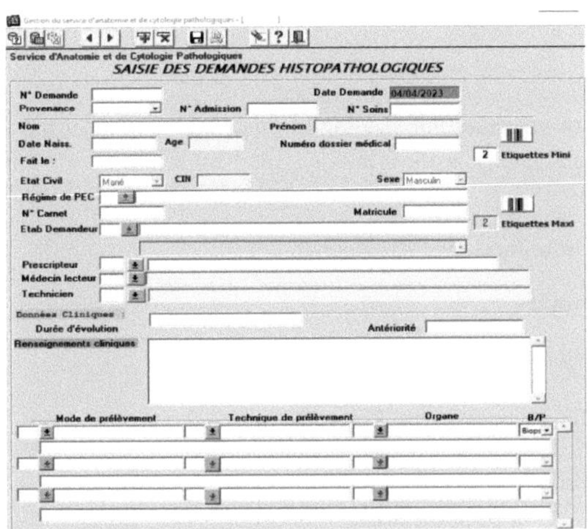

Service d'Anatomie et de Cytologie Pathologiques
SAISIE DES DEMANDES HISTOPATHOLOGIQUES
N° Demande
Date Demande 04/04/2023
Provenance
N° Admission
N° Soins
Nom
Prénom
Date Naiss.
Age
Numéro dossier médical
Fait le :
2 Etiquettes Mini
Etat Civil
CIN
Sexe
Régime de PEC
N° Carnet
Matricule
Etab Demandeur
2 Etiquettes Maxi
Prescripteur
Médecin lecteur
Technicien
Données Cliniques :
Durée d'évolution
Antériorité
Renseignements cliniques
Mode de prélèvement
Technique de prélèvement
Organe
B/P

Figure 11: DMI in the PCR laboratory.

The samples are then sorted according to their type (cytology, biopsy and surgical specimen).

V.3- Labelling

Each sample is labelled with :

- Patient identification.
- The barcode.
- The identification number.
- The type of examination (cytology or histology).

V.4-Transport of samples from reception to the technical room

After registration, sorting and labelling, the samples are sent to the technical room for technical analysis. The technical analysis of the samples is carried out in the following stages:

V.4.a-Study of cells

- **Centrifugation**

The liquid (natural, spillage or wash) is taken to the laboratory where it is centrifuged to obtain a pellet.

• Spreading cells on glass slides

This stage consists of spreading the cytological material using a second slide inclined at 30° to the first, quickly and gently, without pressing too hard so as not to crush the cells.

• Fixing spreads

It is either air-dried or immersed in 95° alcohol.

• Papanicolaou colouring

Papanicolaou staining is carried out in the following stages:

- Harris haematoxylin staining for 2 to 5 minutes
- Rinsing with tap water
- Dehydration in 02 tanks of alcohol of increasing concentration (70° /95°)
- Papanicolaou OG6 staining for 10 to 15 minutes
- 02 tanks of 95° ethanol
- Staining with Papanicolaou Eosine-Azur EA50 for 10 to 15 minutes
- Dehydration of the slides in tanks of alcohol at a concentration graduated up to absolute
- Brighten in xylene
- Eukitt mounting between slide and coverslip
- Reading of the slides by the pathologist using an optical microscope

V.4.b-Study of tissues

- **Macroscopic examination**

The macroscopic examination is carried out with the naked eye, and involves describing, measuring, palpating and then dissecting the samples into small fragments for insertion into cassettes bearing the patient's identification number.

- **Dehydration**

It is carried out in an automatic dehydration and fat dissolving machine (Figure 12). The cycle lasts around fourteen hours. Samples already placed in cassettes are dehydrated by immersion in tanks of alcohol of increasing concentration (70°, 75°, 80°, 90°, 95°, then 100°) for 6 hours, one hour in each tank. This stage eliminates the formalin fixative.The alcohol is then replaced by a solvent miscible with paraffin using 2 xylene tanks for 2 hours. The samples are passed through molten paraffin to fill all the tissue cavities and provide internal support for the tissues for 6 hours.

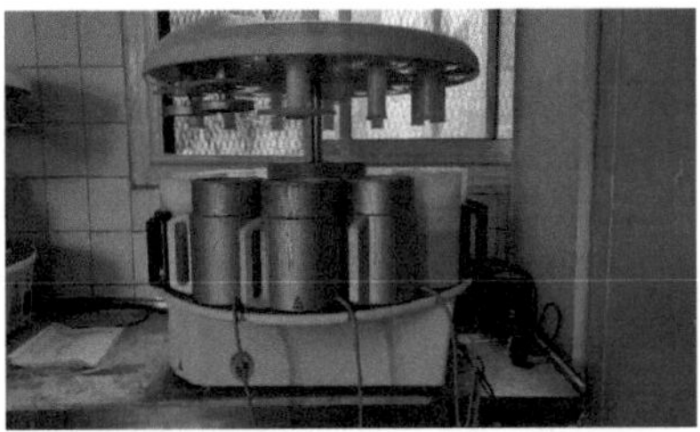

Figure 12: Automatic fat dehydration and dissolving machine.

• Paraffin embedding

This stage is carried out using a paraffin dispenser. It produces paraffin blocks. The inclusion stages are as follows (Figure 13):

◦ Open the cassettes and place the fragments in metal moulds.

◦ Pour in the heated paraffin (59 to 60°), exerting gentle pressure on the fragment to keep it flat.

◦ Cover the fragment with the corresponding cassette bearing the recording number.

◦ Place the blocks on a cooling tray for 15 minutes.

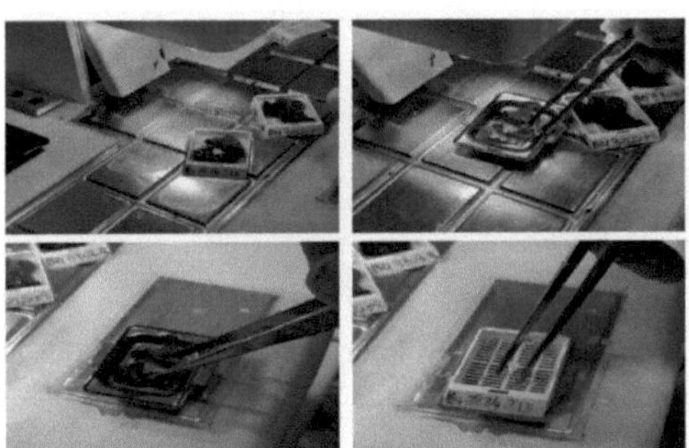

Figure 13: Paraffin embedding

•Planing

This step is carried out using a microtome with a thickness of between [20 and 25 microns]. The excess paraffin is removed to facilitate cutting (Figure 14).

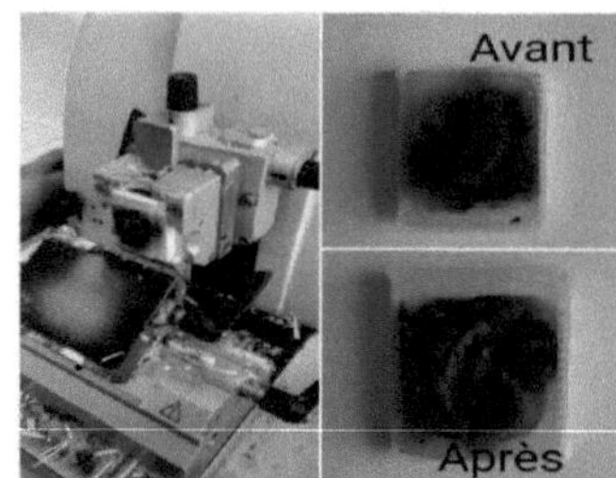

Figure 14: Paraffin block before and after planing.

• Sectioning using the microtome

This stage is carried out using a microtome with a thickness varying between [3 and 5 microns]. The ribbon-shaped sections are placed in a water bath and then collected on glass slides. The slides were then placed on a hot plate (60°) for 15 minutes (Figure 15). The slides were then placed in an oven (58°) for 24 hours for dewaxing.

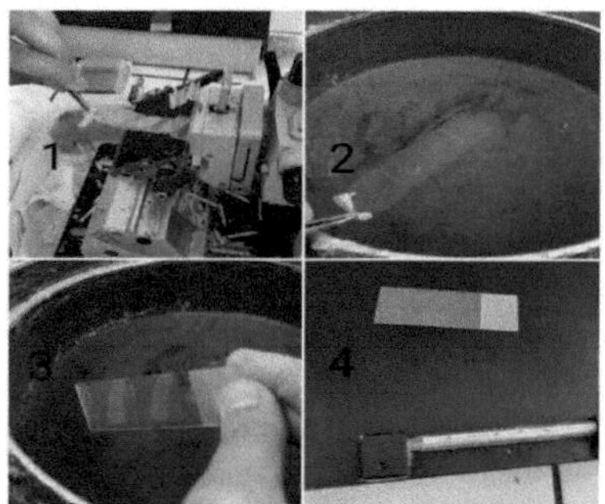

Figure 15: Microtome section.

• Haematoxylin-eosin stain

Colouring is carried out in the following stages. The colouring racks are shown in Figure 16 :

- Passage through 2 xylene tanks for 2 hours
- Passage through a vat of ammonia alcohol (200 millilitres of 95° alcohol + 2 drops of ammonia) for 5 minutes to lighten the slides.
- Rinsing with water
- Hydration of the slides in 3 tanks of alcohol of decreasing concentration (95% to 75%)
- Rinsing with water
- Harris haematoxylin staining for 5 minutes

- Rinsing with water
- Differentiate (turn blue) for a few minutes in a bath of running water
- Staining with eosin (aqueous) for 3 minutes
- Rinsing with water
- Dehydration of slides with alcohol in ascending order (75% to 100%)
- Brighten slides in xylene

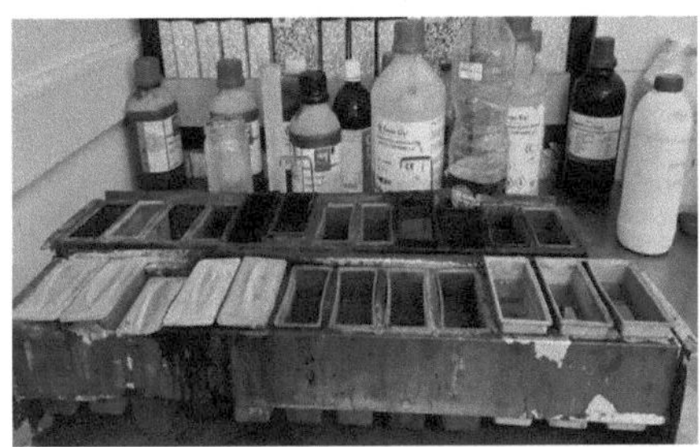

Figure 16: Staining racks.

• Fitting the blades

Mounting between slide and coverslip with Eukitt to protect the sections.

VI. Handling non-conformities

After checking the information on the bottle label against that on the request form and the conformity of the samples, and after technical analysis, the NCs detected were recorded in the NC book (Appendix 4). This was done by indicating the date the request was received, the identification number, the reporting personnel, the type of NC, the cause and the solution adopted.

VII. Improving the pre-analytical phase in pathological anatomy and cytology

To improve the pre-analytical phase in the PCR laboratory, we used the Ishikawa diagram, which helped us to identify the main causes of NC and to implement the following corrective actions:

- Making paramedical staff aware of the importance of this phase by giving them a brochure (Appendix 5).

- Drawing up procedures: procedures describe how an activity is to be carried out in accordance with the requirements of the ACP department.

RESULTS

I. Overall representation of pre-analytical non-conformities identified in the anatomy and pathology department

During the period of our study we recorded 348 cases of CKD out of 36,281 requests for AP examinations sent to the PCR department, i.e. a rate of 0.95%. The different types of CKD are shown in Table III.

Table III: The different types of pre-analytical NC revealed during our study.

Types of NC	Headcount
No request	4
Incorrect patient identification	43
Absence of date and time of sampling	25
Prescriber's signature or stamp missing	32
Lack of clinical information	5
Nature of sample not consistent between card and bottle	1
Discrepancy between application and bottle data	5
Labelling error	10
Number of cytological slides taken not specified on the form	17
Empty bottle	1
Loss of sample	9
Packaging error	11
Sample not compliant with the requested analysis (samples received for a bacteriological examination)	2
Non-fixed direct debit	23
Hyper-fixed levy	1
Insufficient fixative volume	74
Fixer other than formalin	7
Broken blade	5
Routing delays	15
Discordance between the block and the ca	29
Excess colouring	20
Identification number erased during colouring	4
Inclusion error	2
Poor dehydration of samples	3
Total	348

The NC revealed during our study were classified according to 3 categories which are represented by the following figure (figure 17).

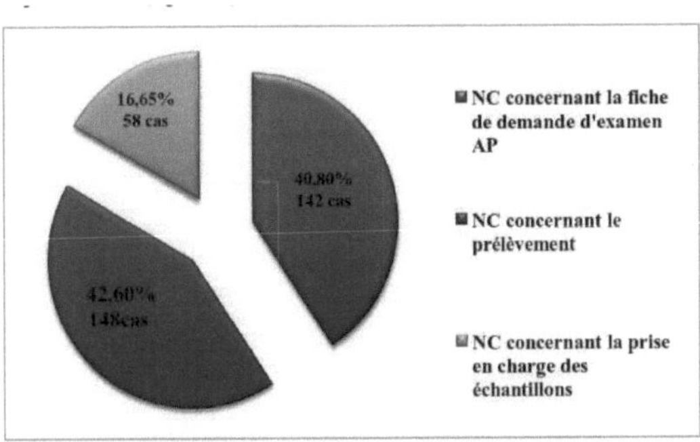

Figure 17: Percentage of NC categories revealed during our study.

II. Representation of pre-analytical non-conformities concerning sampling

We recorded 148 cases of CKD related to sampling (42.60% of total CKD), expressed as percentages in Figure 18.

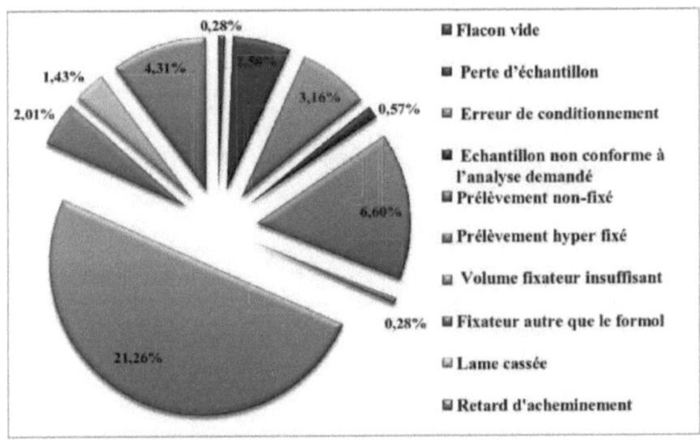

Figure 18: Breakdown of pre-analytical NCs concerning sampling.

Figure 19 shows an example of samples received in the PCR department with an insufficient volume of formalin.

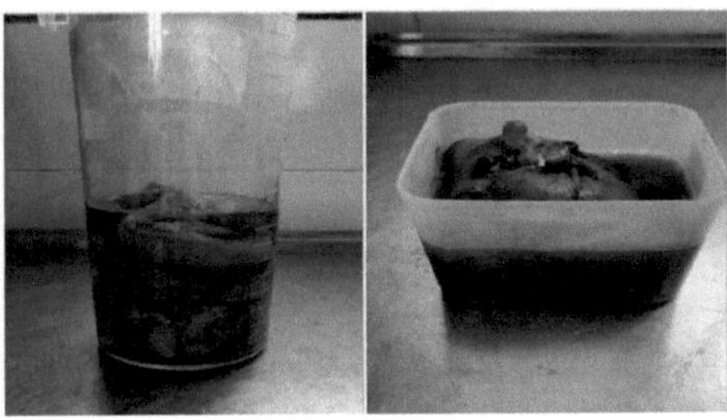

Figure 19: Examples of insufficient volume of formalin.

Figure 20 shows a surgical specimen sent to the PCR department without formalin.

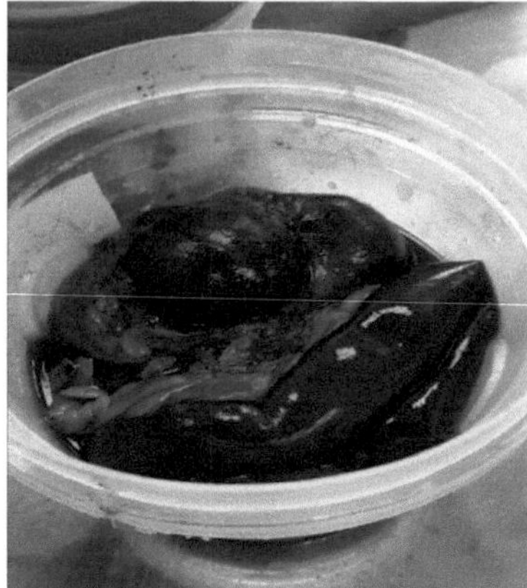

Figure 20: Example of an unfixed surgical receipt.

Figure 21 shows examples of samples sent in unsuitable bottles.

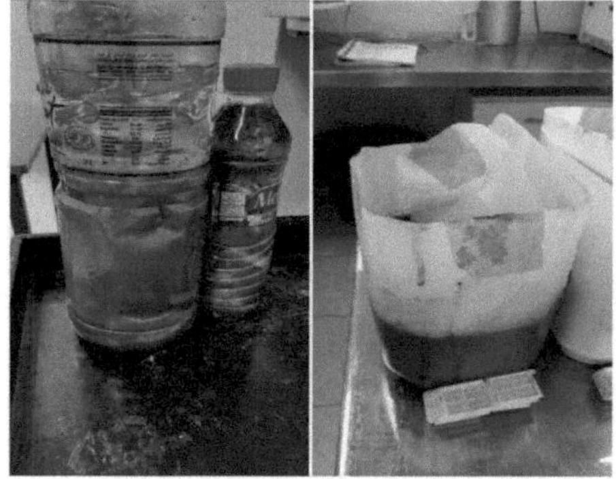

Figure 21: Examples of sample packaging errors.

III. Representation of pre-analytical non-conformities concerning the AP examination request form

With regard to the NCs relating to the AP examination request form, we recorded 142 cases of NCs (i.e. 40.80% of overall NCs), which are expressed as percentages in Figure 22.

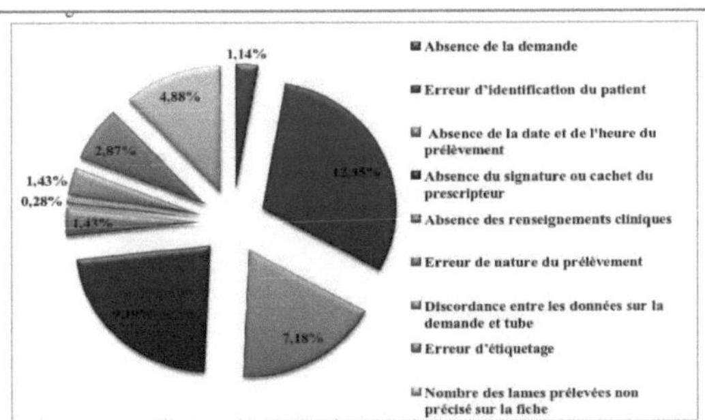

Figure 22: Representation of pre-analytical NCs concerning the AP test request form.

Figure 23 shows an AP test request form without the date and time of sampling.

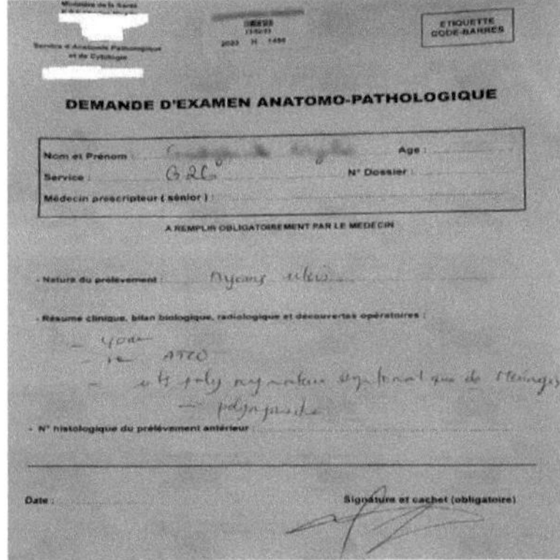

ETIQUETTE CODE-BARRES

DEMANDE D'EXAMEN ANATOMO-PATHOLOGIQUE

Nom et Prénom : Age :

Service : G2C N° Dossier :

Médecin prescripteur (sénior) :

A REMPLIR OBLIGATOIREMENT PAR LE MEDECIN

- Nature du prélèvement :

- Résumé clinique, bilan biologique, radiologique et découvertes opératoires :

- N° histologique du prélèvement antérieur :

Date : Signature et cachet (obligatoire)

Figure 23: Example of a prescription form without mentioning the date and time of sampling.

IV. Representation of pre-analytical non-conformities concerning sample handling

With regard to NCs relating to sample handling, we recorded 58 cases of NCs (i.e. 16.65% of overall NCs), which are expressed as percentages in Figure 24.

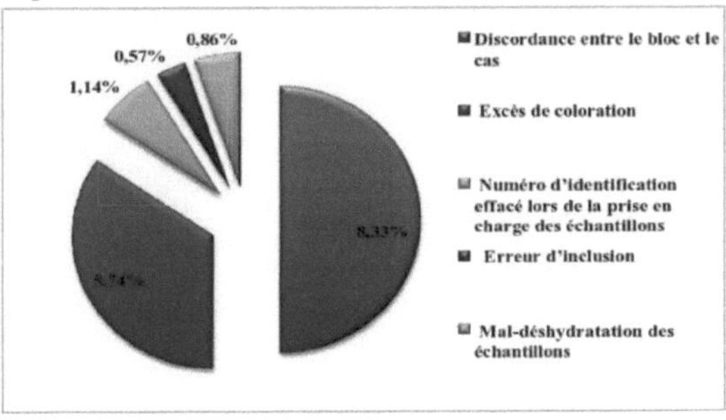

Figure 24: Representation of NCs concerning sample handling.

Figure 25 shows an example of a series of slides for microscopic analysis which are in excess of staining.

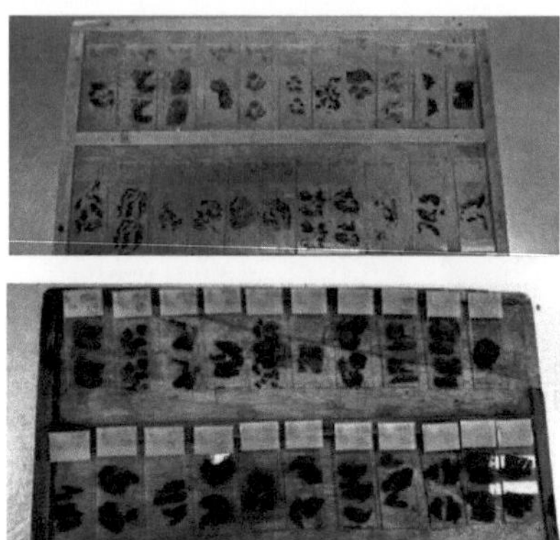

Figure 25 A: series of normal stained slides; B: excess staining

Figure 26 shows an example of poorly dehydrated hard tissue that is difficult to cut with the microtome (excess dehydration).

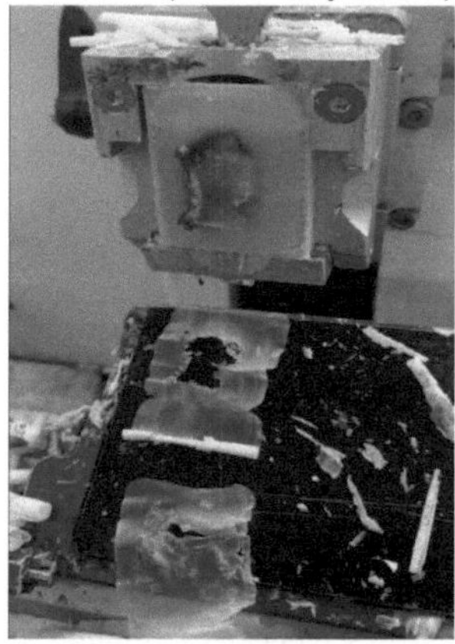

Figure 26: Example of hard tissue (excess dehydration).

Figure 27 shows examples of patient identification numbers being erased when samples are taken.

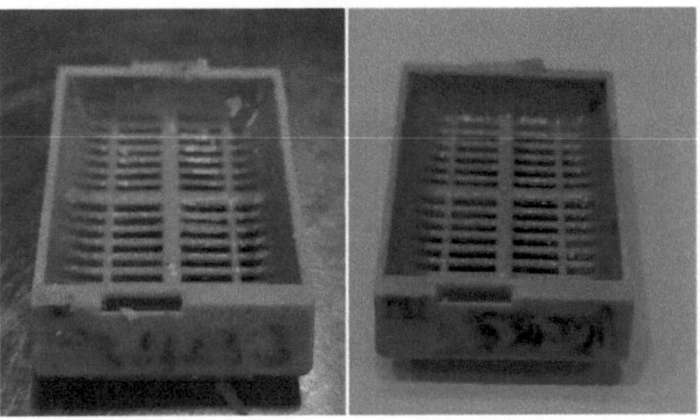

Figure 27: Examples of identification numbers deleted when samples are taken.

V. Breakdown of non-compliances by clinical origin

The various types of CKD revealed during our study came from 14 clinical departments in our hospital. The departments responsible for the CKDs are shown in Table IV.

Table IV: Breakdown of NC by clinical origin.

Department responsible for NC	Number of NC	Percentages
General surgery I	61	17,52%
Obstetrics and gynaecology I	65	18,67%
Gastroenterology	20	5,74%
Dermatology	12	3,44%
Urology	25	7,18%
General surgery II	26	7,47%
Internal medicine II	1	0,28%
Obstetrics and gynaecology II	28	8,04%
Orthopaedic and trauma surgery	9	2,58%
Stomatology and maxillo-facial surgery	20	5,74%
Forensic medicine	8	2,29%
Anatomy and pathological cytology	58	16,66%
Internal medicine I	1	0,28%
Ear, nose and throat (ENT)	14	4,02%
Total	348	100%

VI. Questionnaire results

Our questionnaire concerned 17 staff involved in the internal pre-analytical phase within the PCR department.

V.1- Profile

The questionnaire concerned the people summarised in Table V.

Table V: Breakdown of respondents' profiles.

Profile	Workforce	Percentages
Pathologist	5	29,42%
Resident anatomopathologist	4	23,53%
Reception staff	1	5,88%
Laboratory technician	7	41,17%
Total	17	100%

V.2.-Interpretation of questionnaire responses

V.2.a- Knowledge of the different stages of anatomopathological examination

The responses concerning knowledge of the different stages of the AP examination are shown in the following table (table VI).

Table VI: Breakdown of responses concerning knowledge of the stages of the AP exam.

Knowledge of the stages of the AP exam	Workforce	Percentage
Yes	16	94,12%
No	1	5,88%
Total	17	100%

Figure 28 shows the percentages of the distribution of responses from staff who answered that they were aware of the stages of the AP exam.

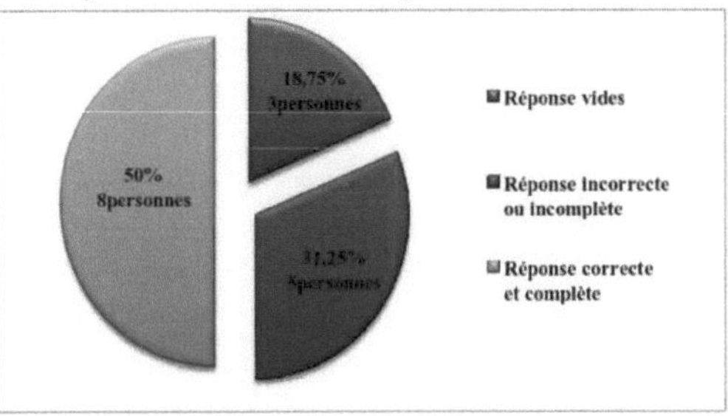

Figure 28: Breakdown of responses from staff who answered that they were aware of the stages of the AP exam.

V.2.b-Knowledge of the stages of the pre-analytical phase in pathological anatomy and cytology

Staff responses concerning knowledge of the stages of the pre-analytical phase in PCR are shown in the following table (Table VII).

Table VII: Breakdown of responses concerning knowledge of the stages of the pre-analytical phase.

Knowledge of the stages in the pre-analytical phase	Workforce	Percentage
Yes	13	76,47%
No	4	23,53%
Total	17	100%

Figure 29 shows the distribution of responses from staff who answered that they were familiar with the stages of the pre-analytical phase in PCR.

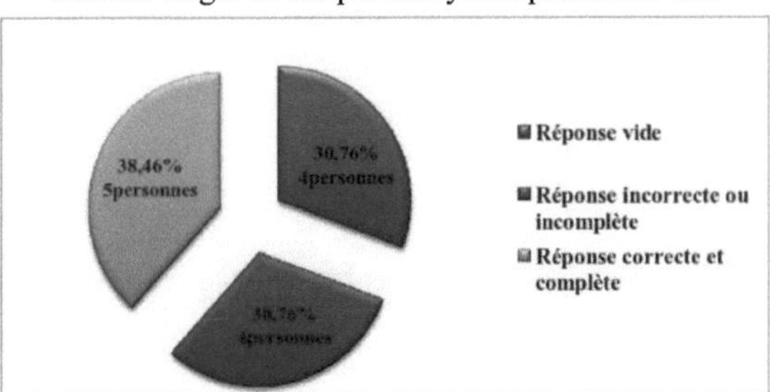

Figure 29: Distribution of responses from staff who answered that they were familiar with the stages of the pre-analytical phase in PCR.

V.2.c-Response concerning the importance of the pre-analytical phàse

The responses concerning the importance of the pre-analytical phase are shown in the following figure (figure 30).

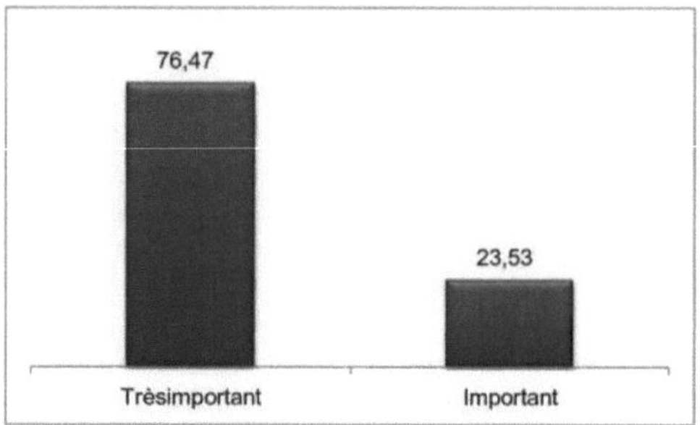

Figure 30: Distribution of responses concerning the importance of the pre-analytical phase.

- Thirteen staff felt that the pre-analytical phase was very important.
- Four staff felt that the pre-analytical phase was important.

V.2.d-Training for the pre-analytical phase

The responses concerning training in the pre-analytical phase are shown in the following table (table VIII).

Table VIII: Breakdown of responses concerning training in the pre-analytical phase.

Pre-analytical phase training	Workforce	Percentage
Yes	8	47,05%
No	9	52,95%
Total	17	100%

V.2.e-Non-conformities

The responses concerning knowledge of a CN are shown in the table below (Table IX).

Table IX: Breakdown of responses concerning knowledge of the definition of a CN.

Knowledge of the definition of a CN	Workforce	Percentage
Yes	14	82,35%
No	3	17,65%
Total	17	100%

Figure 31 shows the percentages of the distribution of responses from staff who answered that they knew the definition of a NC.

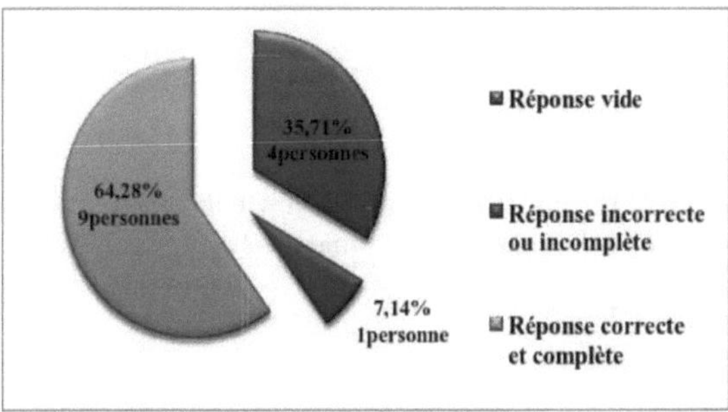

Figure 31: Breakdown of responses from staff who answered that they knew the definition of a NC.

V.2.f-Knowledge of the different types of NC

Table X shows the responses concerning knowledge of the different types of NC

Table X: Breakdown of responses concerning knowledge of the different types of NC

Knowledge of the different types of NC	Workforce	Percentage
Yes	11	64,7%
No	6	35,3%
Total	16	100%

Figure 32 shows the percentages of the distribution of responses from staff who answered that they were aware of the different types of NC.

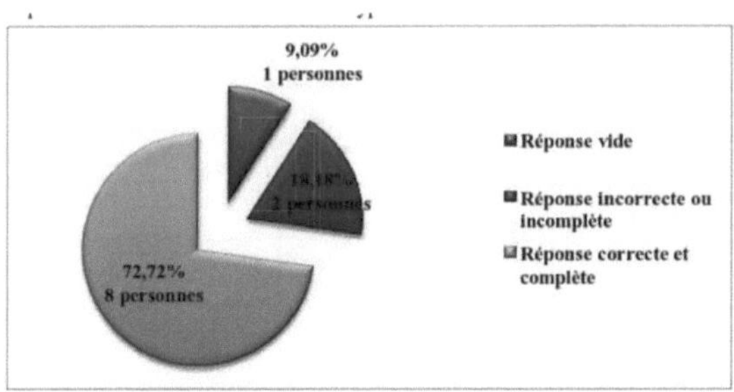

Figure 32: Breakdown of responses from staff who answered that they were aware of the different types of NC.

V.2.g- knowledge of non-conformities that may influence the anatomopathological examination during reception

The responses concerning knowledge of the CKDs that can influence the anatomopathological examination are shown in Table XI below.

Table XI: Distribution of responses concerning knowledge of NCs that may influence the anatomopathological examination during reception.

Knowledge of the NCs that can influence the examination	Workforce	Percentage
Yes	15	88,23%
No	2	11,77%
Total	17	100%

V.2.h- Frequency of recording non-conformities

The responses concerning the frequency with which NCs are recorded are shown in Table XII and expressed as a percentage in Figure 33 below:

Table XII: Breakdown of responses concerning the frequency with which NCs are recorded

Registration From NC	[0%,25%]	[25%,50%]	[50%,75%]	[75%,100%]	Total
Workforce	7	4	3	3	17

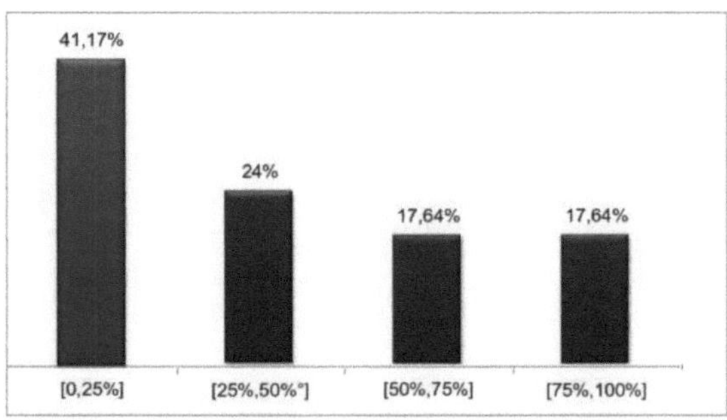

Figure 33: Breakdown of responses concerning the frequency of NC recording.

V.2.k- Impact of non-conformities on analysis results

The responses concerning knowledge of the impact of NCs on analysis results are shown in Table XIII.

Table XIII: Breakdown of responses concerning knowledge of the impact of NCs on analysis results.

Knowledge of the impact of NCs on analysis results	Workforce	Percentage
Yes	10	58,83%
No	7	41,17%
Total	17	100%

V.2.i-How to manage non-conformities

The responses concerning the way in which NCs are managed are shown in Table XIV.

Table XIV: Breakdown of responses concerning knowledge of NC management.

Knowledge of NC management	Workforce	Percentage
Yes	9	52,94%
No	8	47,06%
Total	17	100%

Of the staff who answered that they knew how to manage NC in ACP, 7 proposed solutions and 2 only ticked yes.The solutions proposed by staff to manage NC are as follows:

- The creation of a quality unit within the ACP department.
- Ongoing staff training.
- Drawing up guides and procedures for requesting departments.
- Putting good practice recommendation sheets into ACP.
- Check that colouring products are clean before use.
- Check that the information on the request form and the vials matches on receipt.

VI. Results of applying the Ishikawa diagram to the categories of non-conformities identified

VI.1-5M analysis for a non-compliant sample

The Ishikawa diagram (Figure34) is constructed by considering non-compliant sampling as an identified problem (effect).

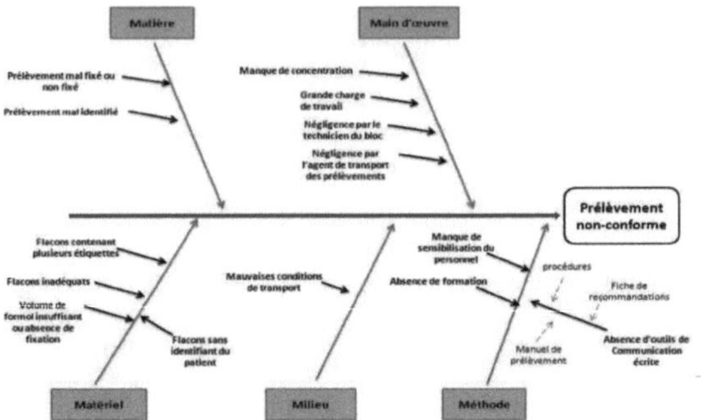

Figure 34: 5M analysis for the non-compliant AP examination prescription form.

VI.2- 5M analysis fora request form for anatomopathological examination

The Ishikawa diagram (Figure35) is constructed by considering non-compliant sampling as an identified problem (effect).

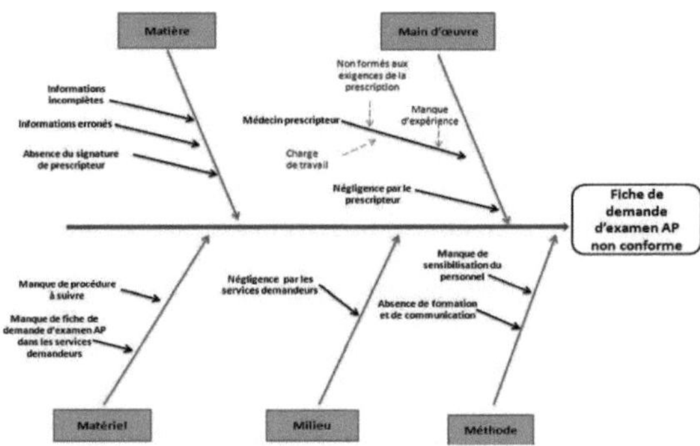

Figure 35: 5M analysis for a non-compliant AP examination request form.

VI.3-5M analysis for a sample handling malfunction

The Ishikawa diagram (Figure 36) is constructed by considering the non-compliant prescription form for AP examinations, the problem identified (effect).

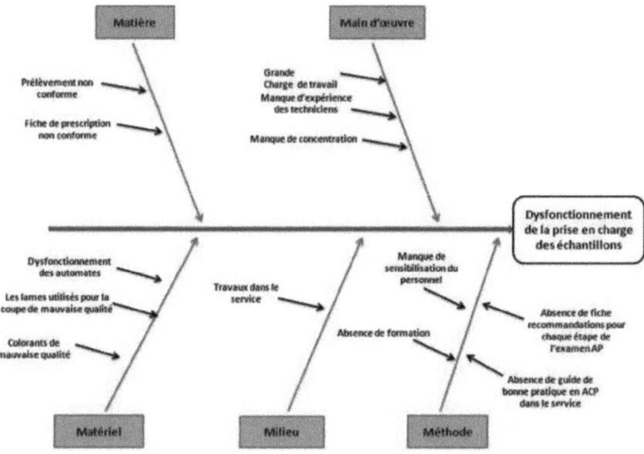

Figure 36: 5M analysis for a sample handling fault.

VII. Brochure on the pre-analytical phase and how to manage NCs

To raise staff awareness of the pre-analytical phase in PCR, we have produced a brochure (Appendix 5) on the pre-analytical phase and how to manage NC. We gave this brochure to the staff who responded to the questionnaire (figure37).

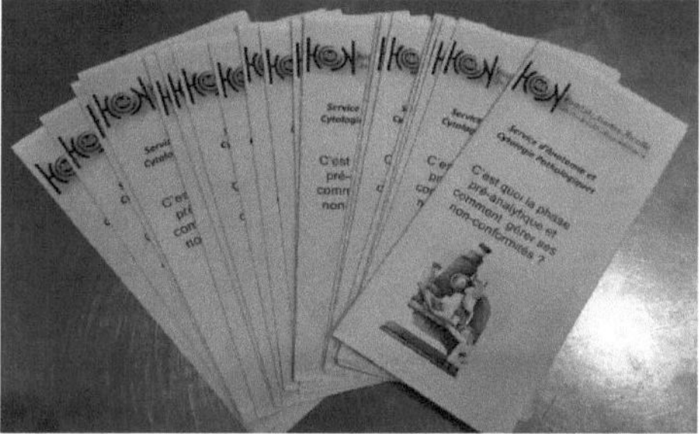

Figure 37: Distribution of brochures to staff

DISCUSSION

Quality in the PCR laboratory is a recent concept [20]. The AP examination takes place in 3 stages: the pre-analytical phase, which is the focus of our study, the analytical phase and the post-analytical phase [2].

The pre-analytical phase is an important stage of the AP examination, which determines the quality of the expected results. It begins with the prescription and ends with the start of the microscopic analysis [3].

Despite changes in sample handling practices, the pre-analytical phase is still the most frequent source of errors in laboratories (85% of errors affecting the validity of test results) [2,15].The aim of our study was to improve the quality of the pre-analytical process in the PCR laboratory. Our study enabled us to :

- Detect the main NCs occurring in the various departments requesting AP examinations and also in the PCR department.
- Assess staff knowledge of the pre-analytical phase using a questionnaire.
- Identify the main causes of NC using the Ishikaw diagram and take appropriate corrective action.

The study was based on 36,281 examination requests sent to the PCR department and revealed 348 cases of CKD, representing a rate of 0.95%. This rate is lower than that of the study by Roque et al, which was of the order of 3.10% [3].

Our study revealed three categories of NC: NC relating to sampling, NC relating to the AP examination request form and NC relating to the handling of samples.

The proportions of the different types of CKD ranged from 0.28% to 21.26%.

NC concerning sampling

With a rate of 42.60%, the highest proportion of NCs were those relating to sampling.

The proportions of the types of pre-analytical NC concerning sampling varied between 0.28% and 21.26%.

Insufficient volume of formalin represented the highest proportion of NCs concerning sampling, with a rate of 21.26%. This may be because the operating theatre technicians were not aware of the concentration and volume of formalin recommended to preserve the integrity of the samples, or because the stock of formalin in each department was not sufficient to fix all the parts.

In our study, 6.60% of specimens were received without fixative and 10% were placed immediately in formalin, whereas in the literature, 0.29% of specimens received without fixative were in the study by Shalinee Rao et al [2]. This can be explained by the fact that the staff were not aware of the importance of fixing the specimens in order to avoid autolysis of the tissues. The packaging error in our study was 3.16%. This can be explained by the fact that the staff involved in the external pre-analytical phase were not aware of the packaging conditions for sending samples to the PCR department. This rate in the literature was 2.27% in the study by Morelli et al [24].

Loss of samples represented 2.58% in our study, which is higher than the rate in the study by

Shalinee Rao et al, which was 0%. This can be explained by the lack of professionalism of the staff involved in the pre-analytical phase.
Empty vials and over-fixed samples represented the lowest proportion of NC concerning sampling, with a rate of 0.28%.

NC concerning the AP examination request form

NCs relating to the AP examination request form represented the second highest proportion of NCs, at 40.60%.
The proportions of pre-analytical NC types concerning the AP examination request form varied between 1.14% and 12.35%.

The patient identification error represented the highest proportion of NCs concerning the AP examination request form, with a rate of 12.35%. The literature showed a lower rate than our study, of around 0.06% in the study of Shalinee Rao et al [2]. This result may be due to the number of requests for examination, which was lower than in our study (around 18,626 over a 3-year period), or to a lack of communication between the requesting departments and the PCR department. The absence of clinical information represented 2.58% in our study, whereas the literature showed a higher rate of around 34% in the study by Sharif et al [25], which may be explained by negligence on the part of prescribing physicians.
The absence of the application form represented the lowest proportion of NCs concerning the AP examination application form.

NC for sample handling

The lowest proportion of NCs concerned the handling of samples, with a rate of 16.65%. This can be explained by the fact that the staff of the PCR department were aware that the samples sent for PCR are irreplaceable and that their handling required a great deal of concentration and professionalism.
The proportions of the types of pre-analytical NC concerning sample handling varied between 0.57% and 8.33%. Discrepancies between the block and the case represented the highest proportion of NCs concerning sample handling, with a rate of 8.33%. This was due to incorrect labelling and the removal of the identification number from the blocks during the technical analysis.Staining error accounted for 5.74% in our study, while Morelli's study showed staining error in 1.5% of cases. This can be explained by the technicians' heavy workload and lack of concentration. The dehydration error in our study was 0.86%; the literature has shown a higher rate of around 1.5% in Morelli's study. [24]
Inclusion error represented the lowest proportion of NCs concerning sample management, with a rate of 0.57%.

Clinical origin

The various types of CKD revealed during our study were received from 14 clinical departments in our hospital. Obstetric gynaecology department A was the department with the highest number of abnormalities, with a rate of 18.67%, whereas internal medicine I and internal medicine II were the departments least responsible for NCs, with a rate of 0.28%. This can be explained by the fact that obstetrics and gynaecology I was the department with the highest number of requests for AP examinations.

Response to the questionnaire

The responses to the questionnaire showed that 76.47% knew the stages of the pre-analytical phase and that only 38.46% specified these stages correctly. This may be explained by the heavy workload and the fact that some staff had not found the time to list all the steps or had not mastered them.

Regarding the importance of the pre-analytical phase, 76.47% considered the pre-analytical phase to be very important and 23.53% considered the pre-analytical phase to be important. All the staff in the PCR laboratory were aware of the importance of the pre-analytical phase. Of the respondents, 52.95% felt that they had not received training on the pre-analytical phase, hence the need for training on mastering and improving the pre-analytical phase in PCR.
The responses to the questionnaire showed that 82.35% knew what a CN meant and that only 64.28% had correctly quoted the definition of a CN. This can be explained by the fact that some staff knew the wrong definition ofa CN, even though they did not know it.
Concerning the frequency of recording of NCs, 41.17% indicated that they recorded only [0.25%] of NCs that reached the laboratory, which represented the major limitation of our study.The low rate of pre-analytical NC recorded during the retrospective study did not reflect the reality of the situation. The NCs recorded during our study were mainly during the training period.

Ishikawa diagram

Based on the Ishikawa diagram, the possible solutions to avoid the causes of NC concerning sampling are represented by the following table (Table XV):

Table XV: possible solutions to avoid the causes of NC concerning non-compliant sampling.

Malfunction	Causes	Proposed solutions
Sample non-compliant	Volumeof Insufficient or no formalin fixing	Inform requesting departments of the importance of fixation and the volume and concentration of formalin necessary for good quality fixing.
	Inadequate bottles	Inform requesting departments that the vials must be of a size appropriate to the size of the room and must be clearly identified and contain a single label containing the patient's contact details.
	Lack of recommendation sheet	Draw up a fact sheet containing the necessary recommendations and distribute it to all departments requesting AP exams

Based on the Ishikawa diagram, the possible solutions for avoiding the causes of NC concerning the prescription form are shown in Table XVI :

Table XVI: Possible solutions to avoid the causes of NC concerning the prescription form.

Malfunction	Causes	Proposed solutions
Prescription form no compliant	Lack of procedure	Drafting of a procedure specifying The prescription requirements.
	Lack of training	Organise training for the staff of the requesting departments on the importance of filling in all the sections of the examination request form and the consequences of NCs on the result and the AP examination procedure

On the basis of the diagram, the possible solutions to avoid the causes of NC concerning the handling of samples (table XVIII) are:

Table XVII: Possible solutions to avoid the causes of NC concerning the management of samples.

Malfunction	Causes	Proposed solutions
Malfunction in the in care of samples	Dyes from poor quality	Check the quality and quantity of Dyes in each tray before starting colouring
	No recommendations sheet for each stage of the exam AP	Draft recommendation sheets for each stage of the AP exam

The strong point of our work was that it was the first study to be carried out in the ACP department.
The limits of our work were :

- The low number of CKDs recorded, as the majority of cases were not registered.
- Difficulties in accessing statistics from the laboratory's computer system to determine the number of examinations requested for each requesting service during the period of our study.

To summarise, our study revealed several factors that are related to NC in the pre-analytical phase in PCR: These factors can be summarised as follows:

- The absence of procedures specifying the recommendations requested by the CPA department
- Lack of staff awareness of the consequences of CKD on patient health

To improve the quality of the pre-analytical phase in the PCR department, our recommendations at the end of our study are:

Recommendations

- **In the ACP department**

- Create a quality unit in the ACP department to ensure quality improvement in the department in general and in the pre-analytical phase in particular.
- Organise quality training for laboratory staff.
- Put recommendation sheets for each stage of the AP exam.

- **Reception**

- The personnel responsible for acceptance must check the following points:

✓Patient identification on the request form and vials.

✓Sample conformity.

✓Compliance with storage and transport conditions.

- Any non-conformities must be noted on the NC register when the applications are received.
- Check the volume of formalin; if it is insufficient, immediately add up to 5 times the volume of the room.

- **In the technical room**

- Check that the identification number on the application form, blocks and slides is the same.
- Indicate the number of slides for each block on the application form.
- To obtain quality colouring, it is important to respect these parameters:
- Quality control of dye solutions before use
- A daily check of the baths (liquid level, order of baths, replacement of solutions, xylene filtration).
- Observe the necessary incubation time for the slides in each staining tank
- Observe the order in which the slides pass through the staining baths.

CONCLUSION

Most AP samples are unique and irreplaceable, which is why it is essential that the pre-analytical phase is carried out according to the rules of the art. A non-compliant sample, even one processed by a competent pathologist, can lead to an erroneous result.Producing a slide for microscopic examination is a complex and slow process, and controlling the quality of the pre-analytical phase will systematically lead to control of the entire AP examination.Our study was the first to be carried out in a PCR department, with the aim of improving the pre-analytical phase and raising awareness among medical and paramedical staff of the importance of this phase.Our study was conducted on a total of 348 cases of CKD out of 36,281 requests for AP examinations sent to the PCR department.The results of our study revealed a low number of NCs with a percentage of 0.95%. Our study revealed three categories of NC: NC relating to sampling, NC relating to the AP examination request form and NC relating to the handling of samples.The proportion of NC concerning the sample was the highest at 42.60%. The proportions of the types of pre-analytical NC varied between 0.28% and 21.26% out of a total of 348 cases.Insufficient formalin volume represented the highest proportion of NCs with a rate of 21.26%.Obstetrics and Gynaecology I was the department with the highest number of anomalies among the departments studied, with a rate of 18.67%.We concluded from the questionnaire responses that 94.12% of staff were familiar with the various stages of the AP examination and 76.47% were familiar with the various stages of the pre-analytical phase.Concerning the importance of the pre-analytical phase, 76.47% considered the pre-analytical phase to be very important and 23.53% considered the pre-analytical phase to be important.Regarding the frequency with which NCs are recorded, 41.17% said that they only record [0.25%] of the NC that reach the laboratory, which is the major limitation of our study.Among the solutions proposed by staff to manage NCs: the creation of a quality unit within the anatomy and pathological cytology department, ongoing staff training and the development of guides and procedures for the requesting departments. Our study concluded with the drafting of a brochure on the pre-analytical phase and how to manage NCs, and the drafting of procedures that are currently being approved by our hospital's quality unit. Human error is never avoidable, but it is recoverable and predictable. Failure to record and/or report a NC constitutes a serious error for the patient's health.Controlling NCs requires staff to be made aware of the importance of reporting any anomaly so that appropriate corrective action can be taken on an ongoing basis. This action must be seen as a source of improvement and encouragement. Close communication between the requesting departments and our department is also necessary, as is compliance with each stage of the pre-analytical phase.

In terms of prospects, quality within the ACP laboratory can be improved by :

✓The creation of a quality unit within the department

✓Ongoing staff training

BIBLIOGRAPHICAL REFERENCES

[1] AlghamdiRS,AlharbiTS,lsubaieWR.QualityStandardssofHistopathologyLaborato ry and Work Facilities in a Developed Country. Arch Pharm Pract. 2021;12(1):90-7.

[2] RaoS,MasilamaniS,SundaramS,DuvuruP,waminathanR.QualityMeasuresinPre- Analytical Phase of Tissue Processing: Understanding Its Value in Histopathology. J Clin Diagn Res. 2016 Jan;10(1):EC07-11.

[3] Roque, Rúben; Henrique, Hermínio; Aguiar, Pedro (2015). Preanalytic errors in anatomic pathology: studyof10, 574 cases from five Portuguese hospitals.Diagnosis, 2.

[4] Jérôme Cros (2012). Means and objectives of anatomy pathology. In general pathologies. Jean François Emile. Elsevier Masson: 1-7.

[5] Raskin RE, Meyer DJ (2010): Canine and fine cytology a color Atlas and interpretation guide W. B. Saunders company 2nd ed, Philadelphia, p 1-17, 231- 252.

[6] ArmelleTassy. Démarche qualité en Anatomie et Cytologie Pathologiques : application à la validation de deux méthodes qualitatives selon la norme NF EN ISO 15189. Sciences du Vivant [q-bio]. 2017. dumas-01885591.

[7] Fayol, H. (1999). Administration industrielle et générale.

[8] AFAQAP. Available on the official AFAQAP website: https://www.afaqap.fr/lassociation/presentation-de-lafaqap.

[9] COFRAC.GUIDETECHNIQUEED'ACCREDITATIONENANATOMIEET CYTOLOGIE PATHOLOGIQUES 2014. Available on : https://tools.cofrac.fr/documentation/SH-GTA-03.

[10] ISO.ORG. International Organization for Standardization [online]. Available at: https://www.iso.org/fr/home.html.

[11] ISO.ORG.https://www.iso.org/fr/iso-9001-quality-management.html.

[12] ISO.ORG.https://www.iso.org/fr/ISO-IEC-17025-testing-and-calibration-laboratories.html.

[13] Guzel, O., &Guner, E. I. (2009). ISO 15189 accreditation: Requirements for quality and competence of medical laboratories, experience of a laboratory I. Clinicalbiochemistry, 42(4-5), 274-278.

[14] ISO.ORG.https://www.iso.org/fr/standard/76677.html.

[15] L.Gendt;A.Szymanowicz(2010).Proposal for the control of the pre-analytical phase according to NF EN ISO 15189. , 36(1), 50-58.

[16] Moen,R., &Norman, C.(2006). Evolution of the PDCA cycle.1-11.

[17] Adda, Fatima; Mansouria Allal, Katia; Beldjilali, Slimane; Betaouaf, Houria; Bougherara, Nadir(2019).Gestion des non-conformités de la phase pré analytique en immunohématologie au niveau de CHU-Tlemcen -Algerie. Transfusion Clinique et Biologique, 26.

[18] Kenett, R.S. (2008).CauseǦ andǦ EffectDiagrams.Encyclopediaofstatisticsinquality and reliability.

[19] Aroubouna,A.B.(2020).Lesnon-conformitéspré- analytiquesaulaboratoirebiomédical de l'hôpital du Mali.

[20] Denis Bouchard(2014).GUIDEDED'ANATOMOPATHOLOGIE.8-88.

[21] Rolls,G.(2012).Fixationandfixatives(2)-factorsinfluencingchemicalfixation, formaldehyde and glutaraldehyde. Leica Biosystem. Wetzlar, Germany.

[22] Anatomopathology, Q.C.C.E.(2011).Guide to quality assurance in anatomopathology: pre-analytical and analytical phases.

[23] orreia, H.M.V., Bernardo, S., Esteves, F., &Garcia, C. (2017).Applicationofstrategies to minimize the error in pathological anatomy. Millenium - Journal of Education, Technologies, and Health, 2(2e), 95-106.

[24] MorelliP, PorazziE, RuspiniM, RestelliU, BanfiG. Analysis of errors in histology by root cause analysis: a pilot study. J Prev Med Hyg. 2013 Jun;54(2):90-6.

[25] SharifMA, MushtaqS, MamoonN, JamalS, LuqmanM. Clinician's responsibility[10] in Pre-Analytical Quality Assurance of Histopathology. Pak J of Med Sci. 2007;23:720.

APPENDIX

Appendix 1

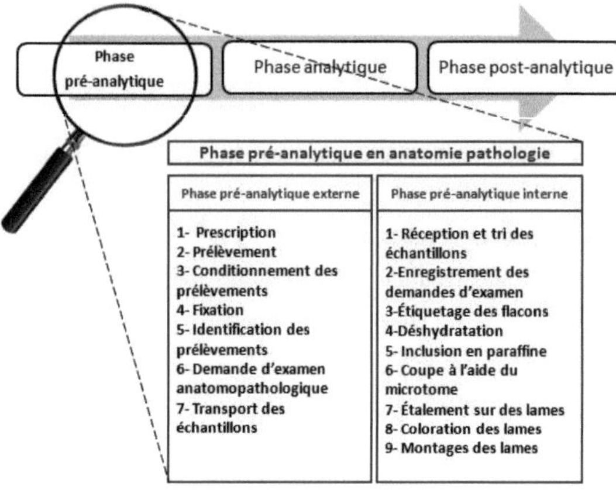

Appendix 2

Évaluation des connaissances sur la phase pré-analytique en anatomie et cytologie pathologique et les différents non conformités commises dans cette phase

Dans le cadre d'une étude concernant la gestion des non-conformités de la phase pré-analytique au laboratoire d'anatomie et cytologie pathologique à l'hôpital Charles Nicolle de Tunis on vous prie de répondre à ce questionnement pour nous permettre d'évaluer vos connaissances concernant cette phase. L'anonymat et la confidentialité des informations collectées par ce questionnaire seront le point de départ de notre présentation de résultats.

1- Connaissez-vous les étapes de l'examen anatomopathologique ?

☐ **Oui** ☐ **Non**

Si oui, citez-les brièvement :

....
....
....
....

2- Connaissez-vous les étapes de la phase pré-analytique ?

☐ **Oui** ☐ **Non**

A quelle étape s'arrête la phase pré-analytique en anatomopathologie ?

....
....

3- Que pensez-vous de l'importance de la phase pré-analytique ?

☐ **Très importante** ☐ **Importante** ☐ **Moyennement importante** ☐ **Inutile**

4- Avez-vous déjà reçu une formation sur la phase pré-analytique ?

☐ **Oui** ☐ **Non**

5- Savez-vous ce que veut dire une non-conformité ?

☐ **Oui** ☐ **Non**

Si oui, c'est quoi une non-conformité ?

....
....

Appendix 3

6- Connaissez-vous les différents types des non-conformités qui peuvent parvenir en laboratoire d'anatomie et cytologie pathologique ?

☐ **Oui** ☐ **Non**

Si oui, citez-les

....

....

7- Au cours de la réception des différentes demandes d'analyse, avez –vous vous trouvé devant des non-conformités qui peuvent influencer l'examen demandé ?

☐ **Oui** ☐ **Non**

8- Est-ce que vous notez tous les cas des non-conformités que vous confrontez ?

[0%,25%] ☐ **[25%,50%]** ☐ **[50%,75%]** ☐ **[75%,100%]** ☐

9- Savez-vous l'impact des non-conformités sur le résultat d'analyse ?

☐ **Oui** ☐ **Non**

10- Savez-vous comment on peut gérer les non-conformités ?

☐ **Oui** ☐ **Non**

Proposer deux solutions?

....

....

....

Merci pour votre coopération

Appendix 4

Non-conformities sheet

Date	N°	Declared by	Ype of non-compliance	Cause of identified / suspected/ unknown+ agent	Solution adopted

C'est quoi une non-conformité?
une non-conformité correspond à la non satisfaction d'une exigence.

Quelques exemples de non-conformités en anatomopathologie

- Erreur de conditionnement

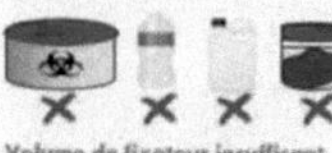

- Volume de fixateur insuffisant

- Fiche de demande d'examen incomplète

-Erreur d'identification du patient

- Numéro d'identification effacé sur les blocs ou les lames

-Excès ou insuffisance de coloration

Recommandations pour gérer les non-conformités.

1 – le personnel chargé de la réception doit vérifier les points suivants:

- ❖ Identification du patient sur la fiche de demande et les flacons
- ❖ Respect des conditions de conservation et de transport

2- Toute non-conformité doit être notée au moment de la réception des demandes sur le registre de non-conformités.

3- Il faut vérifier le volume du formol, si la quantité est insuffisante ajouter immédiatement du formol jusqu'à 5 fois le volume de la pièce.

4- Vérifier le numéro d'identification sur la fiche de demande, les bloc et les lames

5- Contrôle de la qualité des solutions de coloration avant de les utiliser.

6-Respecter le temps nécessaire de la coloration des lames dans chaque bac.

Non-conformités
Actions correctives
Maîtrise

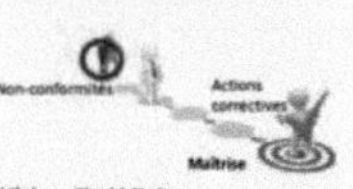

Rédigé par Ghrairi Chaima
Encadrée par Dr Bel Hadj Kacem Linda
Sous la direction du Pr Soumaya Rammeh Rommani

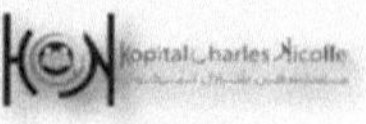

Service d'Anatomie et Cytologie Pathologiques

C'est quoi la phase pré-analytique et comment gérer les non-conformités ?

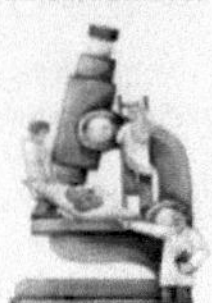

L'examen anatomopathologique se déroule en 3 phases:

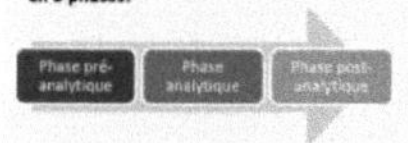

Phase pré-analytique
Phase analytique
Phase post-analytique

C'est quoi la phase pré-analytique ?

Série d'étapes commençant par le prélèvement des échantillons jusqu'à l'analyse au microscope.
Cette phase qui représente 57% (20 % hors laboratoire et 37 % dans le laboratoire) du temps utilisé est à l'origine de 85% des erreurs qui affectent la validité des résultats d'analyses.

Quelle sont les étapes de la phase pré-analytique en anatomopathologie ?

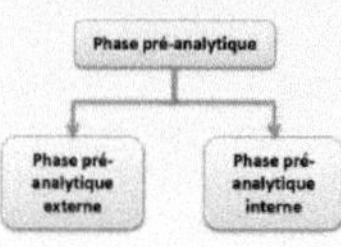

La phase pré-analytique externe: regroupe toutes les étapes qui se déroulent à l'extérieur du laboratoire d'anatomie et cytologie pathologique:

Prescription: un acte médical, réalisé par des personnes habilitées (médecin, chirurgien).

Prélèvement: prélever un échantillon dans le but d'obtenir un diagnostic précis.

Conditionnement: déposer les prélèvements dans des flacons ou contenants adaptés à leur taille.

Fixation: Permet d'éviter l'autolyse et de garder la morphologie cellulaire à l'aide du formol 4% tamponné . Le volume du formol doit couvrir 5 fois le volume de l'échantillon

Identification des prélèvements: L'étiquette contenant l'identité du patient doit être collée sur le flacon et non pas sur le bouchon.

Demande d'examen anatomopathologique. La fiche de demande doit être complète et lisible.

Acheminement des prélèvements au laboratoire

La phase pré-analytique interne: regroupe toutes les étapes qui se déroulent à l'intérieur du laboratoire:

1. Enregistrement des prélèvements dans le système informatique du laboratoire
2. Étiquetage des tubes
3. Examen macroscopique
4. Déshydratation des tissu à l'aide d'une automate de déshydratation
5. Inclusion en paraffine
6. Coupe à l'aide du microtome
7. Étalement des rubans sur les lames
8. Coloration à l'hématoxyline-éosine
9. Montage des lames

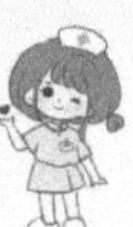

Study of the pre-analytical phase in the pathological anatomy and cytology laboratory

Summary Introduction

Non-conformities encountered during the pre-analytical phase could influence the results of the analyses and have several negative effects for the patient, such as a diagnostic error and/or a delay in treatment. The aim of our work was to detect non-conformities and propose corrective actions to ensure optimal improvement of the pre-analytical phase.

Method

We carried out a descriptive observational study in the laboratory anatomy and cytology department of our hospital. The study was carried out over a period of 3 years and 5 months, from January 2020 to 27 May 2023. We developed a questionnaire to assess staff knowledge of the pre-analytical phase. The main causes of NC were assessed using the Ishikawa diagram.

Results

We recorded 348 cases of non-compliance out of 36,281 examination requests received, a rate of 0.95%. These were mainly errors concerning fixator volume (21.26%), patient identification errors (12.35%) and errors concerning the absence of the prescriber's signature and stamp (9.19%). We concluded from the questionnaire responses that 94.12% of staff were familiar with the various stages of the anatomopathological examination and 76.47% with the various stages of the pre-analytical phase. Among the solutions proposed by staff to manage NC were the creation of a quality unit within the anatomy and pathology department, ongoing staff training and the development of guides and procedures for the requesting departments.

Conclusion Controlling NCs requires staff to be made aware of the importance of reporting any anomaly in order to take appropriate corrective action on an ongoing basis. This action should be seen as a source of improvement and encouragement.

Key words: non-conformities, pre-analytical phase, pathological anatomy and cytology, quality

MIX
Papier aus verantwortungsvollen Quellen
Paper from responsible sources
FSC® C105338

Printed by Books on Demand GmbH, Norderstedt / Germany